Understanding Body Types

- Weight Management Series

Volume 1

Excerpt from Adopting a healthy lifestyle (1-884711-34-0)

Understanding body types
Weight Management Series

C.T. Pam

Published and printed in the United States Innovative Publishers, Inc., Boston, Massachusetts.

Library of Congress Control Number: 2012922836

1-884711-58-8   978-1-884711-58-9 Paperback

Also available in the following formats

1-884711-59-6   978-1-884711-59-6 Kindle
1-884711-60-X   978-1-884711-60-2 Hardback
1-884711-61-8   978-1-884711-61-9 AudioBook
1-884711-62-6   978-1-884711-62-6 iBook
1-884711-63-4   978-1-884711-63-3 Nook

Printed in the United States of America

10 9 8 7 6 5 4 3 2 1   13 14 15 16

First edition, February 2013

For general information on our other products and services or for technical support, please contact our technical support within the United States at pub@innovative-publishers.com online at http://innovative-publishers.com.

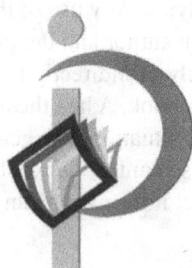

Innovative Publishers

Table of contents

Introduction to Weight Management

With the rapid rate at which obesity has spread over the last couple of decades, the importance of weight management programs has also grown as a consequence. Weight management program refers to all those activities that help an individual to either gain weight, lose weight or even to maintain it at the current level. In any of these goals, a weight management program targets increasing or maintaining the amount of lean muscle mass while decreasing the body fat percentage. Any other way of losing or gaining weight will be unhealthy in one aspect or another and may compromise health in the short term, but definitely in the long run.

Body Composition

Our body comprises of different components, namely fat, lean muscle, water, bones, organs etc. Each of them contributes to the total body weight. For each and every individual each of these constituent elements is present in different proportions. The ratio in which this distribution is present in any individual is called body composition. In the context of weight management, the division is done into two categories – fat mass and fat free mass. A healthy body composition is one in which the fat mass is low and fat free mass is higher. Through different weight management programs it is attempted to alter body composition in a manner that it boosts good health.

There are many techniques and methods to determine body composition. With technological advancements newer and more accurate equipments are available for performing body composition analysis. Traditional techniques such as skin fold measurements are easy to implement but have limited accuracy. Newer technologies such as ultrasound and bioelectric impedance analysis help in doing body composition analysis using simple and portable machines that give extremely accurate results as well. These different methods determine not only the amount of fat and lean muscle tissue but also provide a segmental analysis so that appropriate intervention strategies can be planned as part of the weight management program.

Doing body composition analysis on a regular basis should be included as part of any weight management strategy since it will help in monitoring the alterations taking place in the body as a result of the program. Since the body is undergoing change on a regular basis it is imperative that the program should also change accordingly. A program that was designed for the individual who weighed say 240 pounds will need to be changed when the person loses weight and weighs 200 pounds now. Body composition analysis also provides information on whether the weight loss is happening in a healthy manner or not. In case the weight loss happens at the expense of lean muscle or water then changes need to be done in the program so that these components can be restored to normal levels and fat loss targeted by introducing appropriate changes. A number of new age weight loss methods as well as gadgets are able to provide good results in terms of weight loss but they do it at the expense of good health. Doing a simple body composition analysis will reveal the true nature of these unhealthy methods and systems. Most new technologies also provide information on metabolic rate which is directly correlated the amount of lean mass in the body. Greater the lean mass higher will be the energy that is required by the body to maintain it. The measurement of metabolic rate helps in designing the exercise program as well as the calorie intake required as part of the diet & nutrition plan. Since the needs and requirement of each and every individual are different, the weight management strategy has to be necessarily different as well. Body composition analysis is the first step in designing a weight management program and should thereafter be done on a regular basis.

Problems with adverse body composition

A body composition analysis that reveals high fat percentage in comparison to lean muscle mass percentage points to obesity. Obesity is a modern day lifestyle disease that is essentially a silent killer. It indirectly leads to other physical as well as mental disorders, ailments and diseases that later on deplete the quality of life of the individual and in certain cases may even lead to death. The most common ailments that accompany obesity include type-2 diabetes, hypertension, cardiovascular & coronary artery disease, metabolic syndrome polycystic ovary syndrome and Dyslipidemia. Obesity also leads to gastrointestinal issues such as Cholelithiasis, GERD or Gastroesophageal Reflex Disease, Fatty Liver Disease, Colon Cancer and Hernia; genitourinary problems include erectile dysfunction, renal failure, incontinence and hypogonadism; Respiratory problems include sleep apnea, Hypoventilation syndrome and dyspnea. Apart from these physical ailments obesity also leads to psychological problems that arise from a diminished self confidence and if left unchecked may even lead to chronic depression.

Causes of Obesity

Obesity is caused by an energy intake in the form of diet that is not balanced by equivalent amount of physical activity. The basic law of conservation of energy cannot be violated at any cost and hence, energy excess will lead to weight gain while energy deficit will lead to weight loss. Energy input into the body is through the food that we eat. Energy output is the sum of a number of parameters that include – energy expended through physical exercise, energy spent in activities performed in daily life, basal metabolic rate or the energy required by the body to perform essential body functions such as respiration and digestion; in addition there are a few other parameters such as *thermic effect of food* and *adaptive thermogenesis* that add onto energy output but only in relatively small amounts. It is when the energy input becomes greater than energy output that the body starts storing this excess energy in the form of body fat. Some amount of fat is essential for efficient body functioning but when the fat percentage goes above certain levels it leads to obesity and consequently a host of other disorders and diseases.

This energy imbalance is the objective reason behind obesity but it is important to understand the underlying reasons why this imbalance is created. Imbalanced diet and sedentary lifestyle are the primary causes which get accentuated as a result of numerous personal, social, cultural and familial issues. Genetics and medical conditions also contribute towards increasing the fat mass in an individual. While most parameters seem to be alterable, some of these parameters may not seem to be in control of the individual and a situation of helplessness may be experienced. However, there are ways and means to counter any of these issues that gradually lead to weight loss in a healthy manner.

Genetic factors and Body Type

As mentioned above certain parameters that influence body composition cannot be modified. Genetic predisposition is one such parameter. Genetics define the body type of an individual which then affects the way in which the body reacts to a certain lifestyle and also to any alteration that is forced on this lifestyle. There are different classification techniques for differentiating between different body types.

1. The ancient Indian science of *Ayurveda* uses a classification method based on energy patterns or types. It is believed as per *Ayurveda* that the universe comprises of five basic elements – space, air, water, fire and earth. A combination of these basic elements is responsible for defining the human physiology. The basis of classification therefore is on the basis of energy patterns or *doshas* which comprise of one or more of these elements. The three *doshas* – *vata, pitta* and *kapha* define the person's physiology and all *Ayurvedic* treatments start from the identification of the *dosha* and identifying the imbalance in the *dosha* pattern. Once this is done remedial solution can be prescribed the aim of which is to restore the balance in the elements.

2. The second classification technique is based on the metabolic type. Under this classification technique the basis of differentiation between body types is the dominating gland in the endocrine system. It is believed that the biochemical reactions happening in the body of the individual are influenced and controlled by the dominating gland. This dominance of one particular gland over the others is built into the genetic structure and has a significant impact on the metabolic processes in the body. These metabolic processes take up raw materials such as carbohydrates, fats, proteins in different proportions and occur in the presence of catalysts that are available through micronutrients such as minerals and vitamins. The difference in proportions of raw material

utilized is due to the functioning differences between these glands of the endocrine system. The classification is done into 4 main categories – adrenal (controls reaction to environmental stresses and dangers), gonad (controls reproduction and growth), thyroid (controls metabolism) and pituitary (control the secretion of all glands) depending upon the dominating gland. Different diets and exercise routines are recommended for different body types.

3. The third classification technique and most commonly used in the context of weight management programs is on the basis of Somatotype. The system is based on identifying the association between psychological behavior patterns or temperament with the body structure of the individual. Under this system it is believed that the characteristic behavioral patterns as exhibited by an individual are typical of his or her own body type to a significantly large extent. The body type as in other classification systems is genetically predetermined. People having a similar body type are expected to show similar behavioral traits under this system. The system of classification is on the basis of the 3 elements or Somatotypes that are named after cell groups known as *germinal epithelium* formed during the growth of the embryo in the womb. The three Somatotypes are named after the three germ layers - *mesoderm, endoderm* and *ectoderm* and are therefore called Mesomorph, Endomorph and Ectomorph respectively. Mesomorphs are characterized by a predominance of lean muscle, connective tissues and bone; Endomorphs are characterized by a predominant roundness & softness in the different parts of the body as a consequence of excess body fat; Ectomorphs are characterized by fragility & linearity and are therefore possess frail and weak body structures which are devoid of fat as well as lean muscle. An individual may not necessarily be a pure Somatotype and can be a combination of one or more of these Somatotypes.

These body types are not inflexible to change arising from application of stimulus in the form of exercise and diet. Not each and every one possesses a dream body shape and structure by birth. Similarly, not everyone who has the nature predisposition to a good physique is able to maintain it. The genetic code embedded into our body in the form of body type plays a significant role in determining our body shape but it is not the only parameter. It is true that an Ectomorph may ingest large number of calories as part of diet and may perform rigorous strength training routines but still may find it difficult to add an extra pound of weight. Similarly, an endomorph may perform long duration cardiovascular workouts but still may not be able to shed those extra pounds of fat stored in the body. However, genetic predisposition only indicates the difficulty to create changes; nowhere does it mention that it is impossible. Moreover, in most cases an individual is a combination of Somatotypes which makes it possible to create changes in one direction or the other depending upon the requirement. It is therefore of utmost importance to identify the body type and the goals before designing an exercise program and diet plan. Once this identification has been done, adherence to a scientifically designed weight management program will lead to achievement of the desired targets that have been set.

Components of weight management program

A healthy weight management program should be based on the four pillars of wellness – physical fitness, balanced diet & nutrition, rest & relaxation and mental attitude. A balance between all the four components is crucial for the success of a weight management program. A good fitness routine which is not accompanied by an appropriate diet will not help the individual trying to lose weight. Similarly, a person who does not have the right mental frame of mind will find it extremely difficult to adhere to certain basic restrictions that such a program may impose; as a result of which the whole program fails. A weight management program needs to be customized according the needs and goals of the individual. This customization needs to be reflected in all the components as well. In case even one of them is not in sync it can derail the whole program itself.

Balanced diet & nutrition

A good balanced and nutritious diet is paramount to the success of a weight management program. Not only should it provide the right amount of energy depending upon the goals of the program, it should also provide the necessary micronutrients in adequate quantities for long term sustainable weight loss and overall health. A balanced diet incorporates energy compounds such as carbohydrates, fats and proteins, micronutrients such as vitamins and minerals as well as fiber and water in adequate quantities. As mentioned before the quantity and proportion of the main energy compounds depends on the goal of the program while micronutrients should be available to the body as per standard guidelines such as DV (Daily Value), RDA (Recommended Dietary Allowance) and EAR (Estimated Average Requirement).

In case the goal is to lose weight then an energy deficit needs to be created in a way that energy intake is less than energy output. This may involve reducing the quantities of the energy compounds from the normal diet and vice versa in case weight gain is the goal. As part of a weight management diet plan identifying the calorie content of meals is extremely crucial. To lose one pound of fat, a deficit of 3,500 calories needs to be created. This can be done by ensuring a regular deficit of 500 calories per day throughout the week. A gradual weight loss rate of one to two pounds per week is ideal for the body since it gets time to adapt to the changed conditions. Moreover, gradual weight loss ensures that there is least amount of muscle loss that happens as part of the weight loss process. This is where the efficacy of crash diets or very low calorie diets is questioned. Apart from loss of muscle tissue they cause micronutrient deficiency extremely dangerous to overall health. Certain research studies also confirm that such diets in fact may lead to fat gain since the body experiences starvation and tends to preserve the energy dense compounds for later utilization. This is done at the expense of lean muscle tissue which is difficult to maintain in the body.

In general any meal should include around 55 to 60% energy being provided through carbohydrates, 25 to 30% energy through fats and approximately 10 to 20% through proteins. This principally ensures that while all the energy requirements are met, nourishment of the body is not compromised upon. Even in case an energy deficit is required for losing weight it created in such a way that all nutrients including fats are available to the body for essential functions that need to be performed for healthy a mind & body.

Once the energy requirements have been calculated the next step in the preparation of a balanced diet plan is identification of the meals and meal content. By identification of the meals, it is intended to finalize the meal frequency and the meal timings such that they can be incorporated in the lifestyle in an easy manner. Too many alteration in the existing pattern of life make the adherence to the plan that much more difficult. Therefore, a diet plan should be designed taking into consideration the individual's lifestyle and preferences. In this context the question of meal frequency becomes a pertinent one. The three meal plan has been ingrained into modern day diets since it is conveniently adopted into work life pattern. It may not necessarily be as good and efficient for overall health as well as for weight loss in comparison to a high frequency diet plan such as a 6 meal plan.

Our body requires energy at a particular rate; this rate is defined by our metabolic rate but there may be spikes in demand such as the post exercise period. Clearly, the body does not require energy at the rate at which we eat and the rate at which the energy is released in our body upon digestion of food. In such a situation the excess energy needs to be stored in the body to be utilized at a later stage. The body can do it in the form of glycogen in the liver and muscles but once these limited space stores are filled up then it converts the extra energy into fat which can be stored all over the body. Secondly, whenever a heavy meal is consumed the insulin spike that occurs upon increase in glucose level in the blood, stays on for a longer period of time. In a similar manner this also results in storage of carbohydrates initially as glycogen but later on as fat. Smaller meals ensure that the body gets energy at a rate commensurate to its requirements so that it does not have to convert and store it as body fat. A high frequency 6 meal plan aids in this process of immediate utilization.

The other factor is the proportion of energy that is derived from stored energy reserves versus that derived from food that has been consume in the recent past. The body stores energy compounds like glucose in the blood, glycogen or long chain glucose molecules in the liver and muscles. And fat in the adipose tissue. Whenever the requirement for energy arises the body meets it through one of these sources. When extra carbohydrates are ingested as part of the meal the body stops utilizing the fat stored in the body, on top of this, the extra carbohydrate gets converted into fat. In a high frequency meal plan, the amount of carbohydrates consumed in any meal is limited, which prevents prolonged insulin spike from occurring. This helps in preventing conversion of carbohydrates into fat and also helps in utilizing stored fat for meeting energy requirement.

As part of weight management programs high frequency smaller meals are often suggested due to the aforementioned reasons. The other psychological advantages offered by these plans are beneficial in ensuring adherence during the initial difficult periods of change. By trimming down meal quantities and increasing frequency, cravings that lead to unplanned eating can be prevented. Since, as part of the meal itself there are many meals, the meal content is pre-planned and hence, the chances of eating something unhealthy out of the diet plan are reduce. Uncontrolled hunger pangs are also not experienced since the gap between meals is shorter. This has a dual advantage – apart from preventing binge eating it also helps in avoiding overeating during the main meals. The effect of frequent meals on metabolism has also been seen to be positive in nature. By eating frequent meals, the body is not allowed to go onto starvation mode and thereby the metabolism is maintained at a high since there it is made to experience a near constant availability of food and energy. Increased metabolism helps in burning the extra fat reserves in the body and hence helps in losing weight in a desirable manner. In summary, a high frequency smaller meal plan seems to be much more effective in reducing body fat percentage in comparison to the modern day three meal plan. This loss in fat percentage is ideal for weight loss as well as weight gain. Hence such a meal plan can be made an integral part of any weight management program.

Physical exercise as part of weight management plan

The second pillar in a healthy weight management program is regular physical exercise at the right intensity. It helps in increasing the energy output to create the deficit that is essential for weight loss to take place. In case weight gain is the goal, exercise provides stimulus forcing the body to grow to meet the additional demands placed on it. Whatever the goals may be, like a healthy weight management plan, a healthy exercise routine should include all the components – cardiovascular endurance, muscular endurance, muscular strength and flexibility.

1. Cardiovascular endurance exercises include all those exercises that involve repetitive movement of large muscle groups at a heart rate greater than resting heart rate. Exercises include running, jogging, swimming, cycling, rowing etc. The role of the cardiovascular system is to ensure efficient delivery of oxygen to different parts of the body. Performing regular cardio exercises not only improves the delivery mechanism of oxygen but also helps improve the efficiency of the vascular system and the exercising muscles to take up and utilize the oxygen delivered. Chronic adaptations as a result of cardio activities help in preventing cardiovascular and coronary artery diseases, metabolic disorders such as diabetes and metabolic syndrome and may also help in preventing certain forms of cancer.

2. Muscular endurance exercises help improve the endurance of different muscle groups in the body. Numerous activities of daily life involve repeated movements to be performed of a particular type and therefore utilize a particular muscle group. Improved muscular endurance helps in performing these movements without experiencing too much fatigue in the exercising muscle.

3. Muscular strength is the ability of a particular muscle to lift heavy loads. In daily life, the requirement to lift and carry heavy load often arises but infrequently. If the body is deconditioned to perform such a movement then there is risk of injury. Strength training exercises help in increasing lean muscle tissue in the body as well as improves the quality of

bone health by strengthening them. In such a manner it helps in performing activities of daily life.

4. Flexibility refers to pain free range of motion around a joint. This is one of the most neglected aspects of fitness and as age progresses it becomes the most important component. Flexibility training in the form of static stretches held for moderate to long durations helps in improving flexibility which then reduced the risk of injuries.

All these components of exercise are important in the context of weight management but more emphasis is directed towards exercises such as cardiovascular workouts. These exercises increase the heart rate in such a manner that the extra demands placed on the body force it to rely on stored energy reserves in the body. By careful planning of diet and intensity of workout it is possible to selectively utilize fat stored in the body for meeting the energy requirements. A balanced routine should include 40 minutes of moderate intensity aerobic activity for 3 to 4 times a week, strength training or resistance training of all the muscle groups at least twice a week and static stretching to improve flexibility should also be incorporated at least 2 to 3 times a week. Such a balanced workout leads to weight loss as well as improves overall physical fitness.

Rest & Relaxation

It is important to understand that the actual growth and development of the body does not take place while exercise is being performed. Exercise only provides the stimulus required for growth and development of tissues. The other ingredients that ensure that the purpose is fulfilled are balanced & nutritious diet and rest & relaxation. Post exercise when the body rests and is provided energy and nutrition is the time when the actual growth happens. At this stage the energy requirements should be met from within the fat stores for weight loss to take place. In case this is not done, the body will strip lean muscle tissue to meet the demands post by exercise. Also, in case enough rest is not provided to the body, the chance of overtraining leading to injury increases manifold. Adequate amount of rest and relaxation also helps in maintaining hormonal balance in the body. This is also crucial for healthy weight management.

Mental attitude

A perfectly designed diet plan or a perfectly designed exercise routine is of no use if the individual for whom it is designed is not able to adhere to it. This is where the role of a positive mental attitude comes into picture. Psychological factors play an important role in weight management than is generally imagined. In fact adherence to any plan is solely dependent on the attitude a person carries towards the lifestyle alteration that is being imposed as part of the plan. In case the weight management program is looked at as a set of limitations or restrictions that is forced, the chances of adherence in the short run as well as over a period of time diminish significantly. On the contrary an individual adopting a positive attitude looks at the program as a new positive lifestyle which is embraced with vigour and excitement.

Yoga for weight management

'Yoga' is derived from '*yuj*' in Sanskrit which means 'to unite'. Originating in ancient India, it is a unique combination of mental, physical as well as spiritual disciplines. This union that yoga refers to is the union of the individual with the universal. Yoga is believed to have originated more than 25,000 years ago and contrary to common knowledge it is not just a sequence of poses and postures for improving health and fitness. It is an ancient science that includes tools such as *pranayama* or breathing methods and techniques, meditation also called *dhyana* and finally physical postures or *asanas*.

The modern form of yoga is believed to have begun with Parliament of Religions convened in Chicago in the year 1893. In the convention *Swami Vivekanand* had a deep impact on the thinking of the audience. In subsequent tours in the United States he promoted various aspects of yoga. These talks and lectures led to yoga shedding the tag of a purely religious practice and being accepted by the western world. In the years since then health benefits emanating through regular yogic practices have been researched, documented and published all over the world. It is estimated that in the US alone more than 25 million people practice yoga on a regular basis.

The myriad benefits of yoga include physiological benefits such as improved flexibility, increased strength, better posture, weight loss, effective breathing, stronger immune system, improved bone strength and improvement in medical conditions such as migraine and insomnia; psychological benefits include stress relief, greater awareness, improved energy levels and an overall feeling of inner peace. Yoga is quite efficient in weight loss as well. It advocates a multi dimensional approach that incorporates physical, emotional and spiritual components and does not superficially work on eliminating the symptoms alone. The root cause of the problem is targeted through yoga to deal with the weight problem. It therefore involves detoxification, increasing metabolism, achieving hormonal balance, improving observation & awareness and cardiovascular endurance. Certain forms of yoga prescribe movements done at a rapid pace in a sequential manner that elevates heart rate to moderate or high levels and in such a manner mimic cardiovascular activities. This is very similar to circuit training which is a form of strength training where each muscle group is exercises one after the other without any rest. Such workout principles help in weight loss since heart rate is maintained at a moderate to high level for considerable duration. Apart from the *asanas* that are practiced, *kriyas* such as *kapalbhati* done at a vigorous intensity provides a good cardiovascular endurance workout. Different *asanas* also have different effects on the mind as well. Certain movements performed at a particular pace are known to provide calmness, while other movements help in boosting energy levels. Yoga *asanas* also improve thyroid and pituitary health and balanced secretion of hormones helps in improving metabolism to suit the body's requirements. Other benefits such as reduction in anxiety and detoxification of the body indirectly help in losing weight in a healthy manner. The psychological benefits such as improved awareness and sense of calmness help in immensely improving adherence to weight management program since they bring about a positive attitude towards the entire process.

Meditation for weight management

Meditation refers to the process of reflection and contemplation that helps in calming the mind and in this way relieves stress and anxiety. It has been commonly linked with religion and prayer across many cultures since ancient times. It is often thought of as a tool to improve concentration and as an aid to attaining peace of mind, a path to God and spirituality. Meditation is commonly done by mental exercises that include concentrated breathing, single point focussing as well as chanting. In some cultures it is performed by being completely detached from external worldly contacts while in others the person may interact with the outside world while practicing meditation.

Meditation has developed over centuries and across cultures and civilizations. There is no one form of meditation that fits all the requirements and is ideal for each and everyone practicing it. Which form suits whom depend on factors like state of mind, personality traits and external surroundings. The meditation form that should be practiced is the one in which the person feels most comfortable rather than going after something which is perceived by people in close contact to be most helpful. There is no one single source or authority or text that is referred to for meditation practices. Numerous different forms have evolved over ages each having certain distinct characteristics. A high proportion of these forms though, involve awareness of breath as the underlying platform on which meditation is practiced. Different types of meditation include the following:

1. *Mindfulness meditation* is a popular practice in the West in which awareness of the surroundings is not blocked out. The idea in this practice is to allow all the thoughts to flow into the mind without focusing on any single one of them. This form does not necessarily require quiet and peaceful surroundings and can be performed anywhere. Breathing like most meditation forms is important but is not the primary and sole element. It is a form which is suited to beginners who may find concentrating and blocking out thoughts to focus on nothingness extremely difficult.

2. *Focused meditation* involves focusing on a single thought throughout the practice session. The point of focus can be internal like an imagined object and can also be external in nature like a chant. The emphasis is not on the thought but

on the process of maintaining concentration and not losing focus.

3. *Spiritual meditation* is a form which is closely interlinked with religion and is suited to individuals who offer prayers as part of their daily rituals. The emphasis is on communication and interaction with God and union with the Universal.

4. *Trance based meditation* is an advanced form of spiritual meditation that involves reaching a state of trance by losing self control induced by usage of intoxicating substances. Since the person practicing this form of meditation may not have any memory of the experience, it has a very limited usage, if any, on daily life.

5. *Movement meditation* is a form in which the practice involves constant movement. These movements can be slow & rhythmic in nature such as swaying of the body. These gentle movements are believed to have a calming influence on the mind.

6. *Other forms of meditation* include mantra meditation, transcendental meditation, *kundalini* meditation, *Qi gong* meditation and *Zazen* meditation. Each of them originating in different ages and different parts of the world; differing in the way they are practiced and in terms of their end objectives as well.

Since it is not an exact science, the benefits of meditation cannot be directly and objectively measured. Interest in the scientific community has increased immensely as a result of observations, but studies and research has not determined conclusive proof of benefits derived from meditation. Physical benefits include elimination of stress leading to improvement in conditions such as hypertension and diabetes. The vibrations released are also known to have the added effect of diminishing the negative impact of the disease. Meditation is known to reduce the level of Cortisol and hence reduces stress levels; it also reduces the accumulation of lactic acid which is associated with anxiety. Meditation helps in breath control thereby reducing heart rate and helping the body fight against hypertension; it helps to improve immunity, provides balance to the

15

hormonal system, improves fertility, reduces cholesterol level and helps in weight loss.

While weight loss cannot be directly achieved through meditation it has a more important role to play than any other parameter including physical exercise and diet & nutrition. Meditation does not burn fat in the body but it provides a frame of mind and attitude that is crucial for the efficient functioning of the tools that result in weight loss. Without a positive frame of mind adherence to the weight management program is practically impossible. Meditation helps in identifying the root cause of the weight problem and it does not superficially work on the symptoms of the problem. Even if an individual on a weight loss program is able to achieve weight loss, it may not be sustainable and permanent in case the root cause is not tackled. Meditation helps in improving self control and thereby increases determination that helps in adhering to the program. Moreover, the positive attitude with which the program is adopted magnifies the benefits that may be derived. From the psychological perspective of filling in voids, people have a tendency to go on binges – commonly termed as emotional eating. Meditation helps by working on elimination of desire itself helping the individual practicing it to remain unaffected by the pressures of daily home and work life. The positive attitude that is manifested helps to attain a balance in life. This balance prevents excessive emotions either positive or negative. The person thus practicing experiences an ever prevalent calmness irrespective of the external environment and the alterations that these parameters may undergo. While meditation objectively may not lead to weight loss in the conventional sense, it empowers the individual with a positive attitude – the most useful tool in attaining any weight loss goal.

Meditation also provides numerous psychological benefits. It helps ease stress & anxiety as mentioned earlier. A person becomes calm & composed and is able to visualize the external world with detachment helping in decision making process. Meditation also recharges and provides a feeling of rejuvenation which increases efficiency of all work that the person indulges in. Practicing meditation on a regular basis provides greater mental control that helps in curbing fluctuations in mood and emotion. The spiritual benefits that are derived from regular practice of meditation are manifested in the attitude of kindness and compassion towards others. Union of mind, body and soul leads to an infinite source of love. All these benefits from meditation practice helps produce a balanced personality unfazed by external events and conditions.

Conclusion

For a successful weight management program it is imperative that all these components or pillars be incorporated. When these pillars are not in sync the chances of success of these plans reduces considerably. In fact, neglecting any one of these components may compromise short term as well as long term health and wellness. On the other hand when the wavelengths of the efforts do not match it is very unlikely that the weight management goals are achieved. A positive attitude towards a weight management program that includes a well rounded physical fitness routine, a balanced diet & nutrition plan and sufficient rest & relaxation is almost a guarantee to achieving long term and sustainable weight loss.

Body Type

Body Type

Body type also known as constitution type refers to the various methods of classifying the human body into distinct categories. The systems have either a theoretical or an empirical base. These classification systems help to a certain extent in grouping individuals and prescribing medical, exercise and nutritional programs. Some of these classification systems use body shape as the parameter to segregate different body types into respective categories. Body shapes are generally defined by the skeletal structure of the individual. It also depends upon the amount of lean muscle tissue and fat distributed over the body. The skeletal or bone framework of an individual starts growing at the embryo stage itself even before birth and continues till adulthood, after which this growth comes to a halt. It then remains more or less the same for the remaining lifetime of the individual.

Different Classification Methodologies

Much before the concepts of genetic inheritance came into the forefront, physicians practicing the science of *Ayurveda* in ancient India recognized the fact that these inherited genetic traits are seen in groups. For example, in the current context, an Indian skin color is not expected to be matched with blue eyes of the individual. Similarly, in case genetically a person has a strong muscular build, it is bound to happen that this person shall have a heavy bone structure as well as strong connective tissues to support the musculature. Unlike the first example this is simpler to identify the logical connect in this case. The *Ayurvedic* physicians understood this grouping pattern and developed a medical system which takes into consideration this very understanding.

No one particular exercise routine or weight management plan or even lifestyle pattern can be ideal for everyone. Over thousands of generations we have adapted according to the requirements posed by the environment around us. We have been able to survive by evolving in this particular manner, changing slowly but surely in infinitesimally small steps. Each step is encoded into our DNA. It is the historical account of our evolution. By understanding our genetic type we will be able to understand what works best for us.

Over years of hard work, researchers have been able to develop different classification systems to identify and pin point the common differences between groups of people. Each classification system has a basis for doing so. The initial systems focused on religion, time of birth, race & class as the basis of differentiation. Methods such as sex, blood type, anatomical structure gradually came to be accepted in the next stage of evolution of this study. Most methods of classification may have some or the other form of authenticity, but research scientists over the years have zeroed in upon three methods to make this classification – anatomical, energy and glandular. There is also a definite purpose as to why any of this system does this classification. The purpose may be for understanding the psychology or temperament and categorizing individuals or it may be for the purpose of forming a weight management diet & exercise routine. Each system believes in compartmentalizing according to some basic parameter, although within the category too, catering to individual differences is imperative.

Glandular or Metabolic Types

In the glandular or metabolic method, classification of people is done into various groups on the basis of the gland that is dominant in the endocrine system. Under this system it is believed that in each person the biochemical reactions happening are influenced considerably by the dominant gland. This dominance of one particular gland over others is something that is built into our genetic structure and has an effect on numerous metabolic and biochemical activities happening continuously in our body.

Metabolism is the process by which our body is able to utilize all the raw material that it consumes and convert it into energy and other building blocks essential for the sustenance of life. These raw materials include energy compounds such as carbohydrate, protein and fat, micro nutrients such as vitamins & minerals, as well as air and water. During the continuous metabolic processes happening in the cells of our body these different raw materials are taken up in different proportions indifferent individuals. Some individuals may require more of one particular raw material such as carbohydrates while others may require more of proteins. This difference is created

21

due to the differences in the functioning of the different glands. The 4 glands of the endocrine system that form the basis of this classification methodology are:

1. Adrenal gland controls our reaction to environmental dangers and stresses
2. Gonad controls growth and reproduction
3. Thyroid gland determines the rate at which energy is utilized and the metabolic rate
4. Pituitary gland is the master key and controls the secretion of all the other glands

Certain exercises and foods can stimulate as well as inhibit the secretion and activity of one or more of these glands. Cravings are generally satiated first by individuals and this is what stimulates the dominant gland most. The secretion from this dominant gland affects the brain and manipulates the balance of the body. In case the cravings are repeatedly fulfilled, the dominant gland is over stimulated, leading to imbalance and exhaustion. It may even lead to the gland stopping to function in an appropriate manner. Similarly, in case a particular gland is under stimulated then activities related to that gland may become less prominent. Overall, in both cases an imbalance is created. This imbalance is manifested as physical as well as emotional disturbances. As mentioned earlier, the key to this system is to restore the balance of the body so that all the glands are functioning in a synchronized manner. To restore this balance a balanced exercise program and a healthy diet have been prescribed as part of the system. One has to cut out the cravings and feed on food stuff that stimulates the other glands of the body. Gradually the chemical balance that had been thwarted is restored. Eventually this leads to greater energy levels in the individual and lesser amounts of stress experienced.

Determining the glandular type is done by analyzing parameters such as anatomical characteristics – body shape, skeletal structure, body fat distribution pattern as well as the response that the body gives upon eating certain food types such as energy rich compounds like glucose.

This methodology divides all individuals in to one of 4 main groups as explained above, and each of these groups have certain characteristic traits in terms of physical appearance, diet preference and behavioral pattern.

Adrenal

The adrenal glands are responsible for development of lean muscle tissue & storage of fat; they also control the energy systems within the body along with stimulating appetite. All in all, they help to maintain a balance in the body. The person whose adrenal gland dominates is physically seen to be strong and have a well developed skeletal structure emphasized by broad shoulders and wide chest. They have a strong muscular structure with some amount of fat in the torso, and a large square shaped head. To carry this heavy structure legs are also very strong specifically the larger muscle groups such as quadriceps and hamstrings. Women generally have larger breasts in comparison to other groups and men and women both have buttocks which are generally flatter.

These individuals are stable as well as consistent. They have a clear understanding of what they want and there is significant hunger for power and being in control. This is certainly visible in their healthy appetite and pretty strong dietary preferences. They crave for foods that stimulate adrenal glands include meat, chicken, cheese and eggs. They are attracted towards food that is full of flavor and is rich in content. Since people in this group are prone to putting on weight especially in the abdominal region, the problem with such an attraction is that these foods not only increase the fat percentage in the body but also lead to hypertension, insomnia, constipation, gout and other stress induced issues. People in this category also have a tendency to store toxins in the colon as well as in the muscles which then leads to body pains, as well as digestive issues such as bloating and gas formation.

Individuals in this group should choose new foods that stimulate the other glands as well, so that an appropriate balance is created. A vegetarian diet is ideal for these people, though it may be close to impossible to give up the adrenal stimulating foods altogether.

However, characteristically these people have strong will power and are able to achieve what they set their minds to. Ideally breakfast should not be a very heavy meal and can comprise of cereal, lunch again should be light with lots of greens and some protein, supper can be the heaviest meal of the day and higher protein content in the meal will also ensure that post supper they are able to sleep well. As part of general dietary guidelines people in this group should take care of the following points:

Individuals in this group may find exercises such as playing tennis really interesting and stimulating. The goal should be accumulate some amount of cardiovascular workout and flexibility exercises during the day. Resistance training especially heavy weight lifting is not recommended for such people because of already raised energy levels and that these activities may create a greater imbalance.

Gonad

This particular body type is pertinent only to women. The individuals that belong to this category are very feministic in nature. They have a characteristic pear shaped physique with extra wide hips and thighs with very narrow shoulders. When women become overweight they tend to carry a lot of fat on the outer thighs which can be very difficult to get rid of. Characteristically women in this category are peace loving, warm and nurturing. In general it has been experienced that women with this body type are not pro competition but may actually stand up for anything that they strongly believe in.

The types of food that attract people in this group are creamy as well as spicy foods that stimulate the gonad or sex glands. The rich food leads to accumulation of fat, but this takes place at a slightly slower rate. They find it difficult to break down fat molecules in food and this leads to quite a bit of imbalance. Fatigue and nausea are often experienced after a heavy meal. They are prone to issues such as arthritis, allergies, kidney and gall bladder problems, and issues with female sex organs. These issues come about since the body is not able to break the fat down and it gets stored as toxins within the system. People in this group should therefore avoid fried foods such as chips, spices, sugar, cream, organ meat and caffeine.

Breakfast should be light and can include fruits along with a little lean protein source. Lunch should consist of fresh salads without any creamy dressings. The dominant sex glands as can be expected are active during the night and this when the largest protein meal should be consumed. However, care needs to be taken that the meal is not very heavy otherwise sleep gets disturbed for people in this group. A general rule that is even more pertinent in case of this group is that enough water should be consumed between the meals.

The exercises that can be taken up include cardiovascular activities such as running and jogging, as well as aerobic activities that work on the lower body. Activities such as gymnastics are also recommended for this group since they tend to work on creating a balance between the lower and upper halves of the body, which is an issue that this group faces.

Pituitary

Individuals in this category are generally considered soft, with distributed baby fat all over the body. Females generally have smaller hips and breasts. Males in this group seem to possess large heads in comparison to the rest of the body framework. Characteristically, individuals in this group are the least physical in nature. Individuals in this category are the ones who did not develop physically at a pace at which others did. They appear lost and dreamy and enjoy activities that stimulate the mind. These include the philosophers and researchers who can produce dramatic pieces of work if given an opportunity to work without much disturbance.

The digestive system is generally weak and therefore cravings are for foods that are light such as milk, yogurt and cheese. Apart from a particular liking for these foods, there is an attraction for other foods such as simple & complex carbohydrates. Eating of dairy products as mentioned before, stimulates the pituitary gland. Over stimulation can lead to allergies, gastrointestinal & colon related problems and skin conditions. People in this group also do not reach physical maturity fast and may also face many sex related problems, this is a direct result of issues with the pituitary gland. To create balance, in case a dietary change is required such as substituting dairy products with other foods, this group finds it the easiest to incorporate such a change. Increasing the protein intake as part of the diet is also extremely crucial. This protein should essentially come from non-dairy sources only. People in this group should try and consume a heavy breakfast as well as a heavy lunch while keeping the dinner light. All three meals should incorporate a high percentage of protein from a variety of sources other than dairy products.

Activities such as martial arts, yoga, tai chi and dance are recommended. Regular activities such as walking become monotonous and people in this group tend to think of other things while performing these mechanical movements. It is therefore preferred that an activity that requires a higher level of concentration is chosen to be performed on a regular basis.

Thyroid

The Thyroid gland is responsible for ensuring a stable metabolic rate in the body. The physical characteristics of individuals in this group include wide shoulders and narrow hips which is characteristically a swimmer's physique. They have a tendency to add on fat around the chest and torso. Thyroid glands are very erratic in nature, and therefore the people in whom this is the dominating gland: naturally have numerous mood fluctuations. They can exhibit immense lethargy at one point in time and at another they could be bursting with energy with the aim to produce something creative. Professions such as art & music are suitable for such individuals with high latent capacity for quality creative work.

Stimulating food for thyroid gland include simple sugars as well as complex carbohydrates. As is expected craving and satiation leads to overstimulation of the thyroid glands causing numerous issues. It is therefore best for people in this group to avoid foods such as white flour, sugar, fruit juices, bread, pasta and fried carbohydrates such as wafers and chips. Ideal replacements are foods that are high in protein such as lean meats such as chicken, fish and eggs. Caffeine should be replaced by green teas.

Exercises such as swimming as well as aerobic activities that are low impact in nature performed at least 3 times a week seem to be ideally suited to people in this group. Strenuous exercises that increase the heart rate over a certain level and maintain it there, are also not recommended since fatigue, exhaustion and energy swings are extremely common within this group. The intensity can be increased gradually once adherence to the exercise program is not under question.

It is important to understand that the glandular type or metabolic type of the body determines the ideal ratio in which macro nutrients should be consumed in the food. The theory clearly explains the reason for cravings and the need to curb the cravings. Over stimulating as well as under stimulating of the certain glands in the body creates an imbalance which then leads to health disorders. It is therefore important to correct this imbalance as soon as possible. This can be done through a properly designed exercise and diet program.

Energy Types

Classification on the basis of energy type is the oldest classification technique based on the ancient science of *Ayurveda* that originated in India. The classification is done on the basis of energy patterns, also called *doshas*. In *Ayurveda* it is believed that physical matter itself is largely made up of nothing with energy waves. The duality of particle and wave is understood by modern science today and the interaction between physical matter and energy waves was exactly the basis on which *Ayurveda* was practiced even in those ancient times. The field of medicine on the current date is beginning to study the interactions that exist between the endocrine system, central and peripheral nervous system and the immune system. The mode in which this communication takes place between the systems is not very clear but is evident that chemicals such as neuro-transmitters are utilized by the brain which is a part of the central nervous system, to do this communication.

In *ayurveda*, the universe is composed of five fundamental elements – *akasha* or space, *vayu* or air, *agni* or fire, *apu* or water *and prithvi* or earth. It is believed that human physiology like the universe is also composed of these five elements. The three *doshas* or biological humors are called *vata, pitta* and *kapha*. Each of them is a com-

27

bination of two elements from the set of five constituent elements of the universe. *Vata or wind* is a combination of air and space, *pitta or bile* is a combination of water and fire and finally *kapha or phlegm* is a combination of earth and water. *Vata* controls movement both in the mind and the body; *pitta* regulates metabolic activities and finally *kapha* which is responsible for the structure. Each of these *doshas* has its sub-types and the combination of these *doshas* that we inherit at birth is responsible for everything that happens within us. Together these 3 *doshas* achieve a state of harmony in all aspects of our life when they are present in equal quantities thus being able to create a balance. When this balance is disturbed it gets manifested in various unhealthy ways.

Each individual has the three *doshas* in a particular proportion. This is similar to being ingrained in our genetic code. This combination of *doshas* is said to be *prakriti* and is different for each individual. It is uncommon to have all three *doshas* in equal proportions; generally each individual will have a combination of 2 dominant *doshas* and one which is not. Specifically there are 10 possible combinations for the *prakriti* of an individual. These are as following:

1. *Vata – prakriti* in which *vata* is dominant over other two doshas

2. *Pitta – prakriti* in which *pitta* is dominant over other two doshas

3. *Kapha – prakriti* in which *kapha* is dominant over other two doshas

4. *Vata – Pitta – prakriti* in which *vata & pitta* are the two dominant *doshas* with *vata* overriding *pitta*

5. *Pitta – Vata – prakriti* in which *pitta & vata* are the two dominant *doshas* with *pitta* overriding *vata*

6. *Vata – Kapha – prakriti* in which *vata & kapha* are the two dominant *doshas* with *vata* overriding *kapha*

7. *Kapha – Vata – prakriti* in which *kapha & vata* are the two dominant *doshas* with *kapha* overriding *vata*

8. *Pitta – Kapha – prakriti* in which *pitta & kapha* are the two dominant *doshas* with *pitta* overriding *kapha*

9. *Kapha – Pitta – prakriti* in which *kapha & pitta* are the two dominant *doshas* with *kapha* overriding *pitta*

10. *Vata – Pitta – Kapha – prakriti* in which there is a balance between the three *doshas*

As was the case in glandular system of classification, in *ayurveda* too, all the three *doshas* influence each and every individual but one particular *dosha* may be dominant as described above. It is believed in *ayurveda* that all ailments arise as a result of imbalance that is created in the *doshas*. The first step therefore, in any *ayurvedic* treatment plan is to identify the *prakriti* of the person. An *ayurvedic* physician does so by assessing the pulse of the person and under-standing the imbalance in the body and the reason behind it. Only after this assessment, a treatment plan can be suggested to restore the balance.

By balance it needs to be clarified at this stage, it is meant that the original *prakriti* is maintained. This is essential for leading a good, healthy life. However, due to our lifestyle choices, dietary habits, choice of environment that we live in, nature of our relations with other people, a decrease or increase in one of the *doshas* may happen leading to movement away from *prakriti* and consequently causing an imbalance. It is because of this very reason that the aim of any *ayurvedic* treatment plan is always to restore the balance.

Vata Dosha

The characteristics of *vata dosha* include cool, lacking weight, dry, rough, tiny penetrating particles, moving continuously, unlimited and unbounded. Individuals with *vata* in their *prakriti* have a thin and wiry skeletal structure; have voluminous hair and skin that is dry. In terms of their behavior they are lively, quick in thought and action, are good speakers and are affable and therefore make friends easily. These individuals are extremely creative and their level of enthusiasm is generally very high. They sleep very light and prefer warmer climates.

Generally, people who have a dominant *vata* will exhibit the characterics as mentioned above. However, issues arise when *vata* characteristics become aggravated beyond a certain level, creating an imbalance. Similarly, an imbalance is created when a person with *pitta* or *kapha* dominant *dosha* start exhibiting *vata* characteristics. This again is a sign of imbalance and needs to be corrected. The signs and symptoms that suggest a *vata* imbalance include constant tension and anxiousness, feeling of fatigue, restless sleep, dry and flaking skin, brittle hair with split ends, chapped lips and sore throat, indigestion, gas build up, limited attention span with tendency to keep on working and moving. The reasons for a *vata* imbalance can be consumption of extremely cold beverages, eating raw food, eating extremely dry food, exposure to cold conditions, travel exertions and increased stress levels.

Correction can be done through lifestyle changes such as following a *vata* balancing dietary routine as suggested by an *ayurvedic* physician. In *ayurveda* as a general practice, antidotes are generally exactly opposite to the problem. For example, to counter *vata* characteristic of dryness, include foods that are liquid in nature; to counter roughness, include soft foods; to counter the cold foods that are warm should be consumed. The following list includes tips on balancing *vata* through diet:

1. Food should be cooked and eaten when warm. Cooked cereals, vegetable soups and beverages such as almond milk should be consumed. Raw foods such as salads and sprouts should be avoided

2. Food should not be dry, therefore small quantities of clarified butter should be used for heating and olive oil should be used when needed as a dressing. Cooked foods such as grains and baked vegetables can be consumed. Dry foods such as cereals and crackers should be avoided

3. Foods that can be consumed include vegetables such as carrots, bottle gourd, beetroot and green leafy vegetables such as spinach; basmati rice and whole wheat Indian flat breads.

4. Nuts are good *vata* balancers. Almonds can be soaked at night and consumed in the morning. Other nuts such as cashews and walnuts can also be consumed.

5. Spices aide digestion and also have a warming effect. Combination of spices can be used for preparation of all dishes

6. A combination of salty, sour and sweet help in balancing *vata*. Therefore, all three tastes should be included as part of daily meal plan. Citrus fruits, dried fruit, salted nuts can be consumed. Bitter and pungent tasting foods should be avoided.

7. Warm water should be consumed at regular intervals throughout the day

The following list includes tips on lifestyle that help in balancing *vata:*

1. Meals should never be skipped. In fact the meals should also be consumed in a peaceful manner and not in a hurry while on the move.

2. *Vata dosha* is characterized by restlessness and continuous movement in an irregular and uncontrolled manner. The first shift should be towards a more manageable lifestyle routine with regular timings for most activities such as waking up, sleeping and eating.

3. Getting up early after adequate amount of rest and walking for at least 30 minutes on a daily basis helps in balancing *vata*

4. At least 30 minutes should be devoted to practice of meditation on a daily basis. It has a calming and soothing influence and helps in overcoming the restlessness that is so characteristic of a *vata* dominant individual

5. To take care of dry skin and to improve blood circulation an *ayurvedic* massage should be taken before shower or bath. Jojoba oil or almond oil can be used for the massage.

6. Body should be protected from the cold, and warm clothing should be worn whenever one moves outdoors.

Pitta Dosha

As mentioned in the previous section, *Pitta* is a combination water and fire. The characteristics of *pitta* include sharp, hot, burning, acidic, pungent, liquid, flowing in an uncontrolled manner. Individuals with *pitta* dominant *prakriti* have a medium sized skeletal structure, have thin hair with signs of thinning and premature graying and have a sensitive warm and fair skin. They are sharp and very determined in their approach towards things. They are extremely ambitious and have a purpose about everything that they do. Self confidence is extremely high and they also possess an entrepreneurial spirit. All these are typical signs of a *pitta* dominant *prakriti* of an individual.

Generally, people who have a dominant *pitta* will exhibit the characteristics as mentioned above. However, issues arise when *pitta* characteristics become aggravated beyond a certain level, creating an imbalance. Similarly, an imbalance is created when a person with *vata* or *kapha* dominant *dosha* start exhibiting *pitta* characteristics. This again is a sign of imbalance and needs to be corrected. The signs and symptoms that suggest a *pitta* imbalance include constant irritation and impatience, obsession with work, acidity and heartburn, sensitive skin, feeling warm and uncomfortable even when indoors, regular involvement in arguments, short temper and sarcasm as a part of speech.

As was the case with *vata,* restoration of balance can be done through lifestyle changes such as following a *pitta* balancing dietary routine as suggested by an *ayurvedic* physician. For example, to counter the liquid nature of *pitta*, include heavy foods that are dry in nature; to counter the heat foods that are cool should be consumed. The following list includes tips on balancing *pitta* through diet:

1. Foods that have a cooling effect are ideal for *pitta* balancing. These include fresh and juicy fruits such as pear, milk, almonds, dates and coconut

2. Foods that can be eaten include dry substances such as crackers, dry cereal, granola bars; vegetables such as carrots, asparagus, green leafy vegetables, cauliflower, broccoli and beans; basmati rice and whole wheat Indian flat breads.

They are even better when consumed with *pitta* pacifying spices and chutneys. Other grains such as amaranth and oats can also be consumed.

3. Clarified butter should be utilized for cooking purposes since it is understood to cool both mind and body.

4. To aid in digestion buttermilk can be consumed along with meals and water consumed should be cool.

5. A combination of astringent, bitter and sweet help in balancing *pitta*. Therefore, all three tastes should be included as part of daily meal plan. Milk, soaked almonds, ripened fruits can be consumed. Salty and pungent tasting foods should be avoided.

6. Spices need to be chosen carefully so that they are not too hot and pungent. Spices such as turmeric, coriander, cumin, fennel and cinnamon can be consumed in small quantities.

The following list includes tips on lifestyle that help in balancing *pitta:*

1. To balance *pitta* one should first and foremost be cool, both emotionally and physically. Avoid getting out in the sun, on an empty stomach or even after having a sour or spicy meal.

2. At least 30 minutes should be devoted to practice of meditation on a daily basis. It helps to balance the emotions and helps to create harmony between mind, body and soul.

3. Since skin is sensitive, an *ayurvedic* massage would be immensely beneficial each day before a bath. For the purpose coconut oil should be used and a couple of drops of aromatic essential oils such as rose can be added.

4. No meal should be skipped. Breakfast and lunch should be relatively heavier in comparison to dinner which should be kept light. Skipping meals means there is a huge gap between two meals and that will result in acidity.

5. It is important to break the obsession that one has with work. A recreation activity should be an everyday affair, even though it may be for a small duration.

33

6. Protection from the sun and heat is important. In case one has to move out in the sun, wearing loose cotton clothing, using sun glasses and drinking plenty of water is imperative

Kapha Dosha

Kapha is a combination earth and water. The characteristics of *kapha* include sweet, stability, cold, soft, lubricating, unctuous and slippery. Individuals with *kapha* dominant *prakriti* have a large sized skeletal structure, thick & oily skin, wavy and thick set hair. They are extremely calm and stable, in speech as well as in thought. They are very loyal by nature and have a kind of serenity about them. They are heavy sleepers and feel very uncomfortable in clammy and wet environments. Their disposition is sweet and calm and a feeling of peace and comfort is experienced around them. All these are typical signs of a *kapha* dominant *prakriti* of an individual.

Generally, people who have a dominant *kapha* will exhibit the characteristics as mentioned above. However, issues arise when *kapha* characteristics become aggravated beyond a certain level, creating an imbalance. Similarly, an imbalance is created when a person with *vata* or *pitta* dominant *dosha* start exhibiting *kapha* characteristics. This again is a sign of imbalance and needs to be corrected. The signs and symptoms that suggest a *kapha* imbalance include easily gaining weight, fatigue and exhaustion despite no strenuous activity being performed, difficulty in waking up even after prolonged sleep, oily skin, oily hair, feeling of heaviness and congestion, slow digestion rate, lethargy and lack of motivation.

As was the case with *pitta,* restoration of balance can be done through lifestyle changes such as following a *kapha* balancing dietary routine as suggested by an *ayurvedic* physician. For example, to counter the oily nature of *kapha,* include foods that are dry in nature; to counter the heaviness, foods that are light but nourishing should be consumed; to counter the cold and sweet characteristics of *kapha* warm foods which have a tangy and spicy taste should be consumed. The following list includes tips on balancing *kapha* through diet:

1. Oily foods should be avoided. Clarified butter should be utilized for cooking purposes but only in very small quantities. Food should ideally be steamed or boiled along with spices heated in a little clarified butter for taste.

2. Light but foods that warm have a *kapha* balancing nature. These include vegetable soups, stews, dals, and combination of vegetables with some grains. Salt should be avoided, and as a substitute herbs and spices can be added for flavor.

3. A combination of astringent, bitter and pungent help in balancing *kapha*. Therefore, all three tastes should be included as part of daily diet. Apples, beans, cauliflower, broccoli are ideal. Sweet, sour and salty food dishes should be avoided as much as possible

4. Foods that can be eaten include dry substances such as low salt crackers, dry rice cakes; lighter grains such as millet and barley are ideal ; vegetables such as carrots, okra, asparagus, green leafy vegetables, cauliflower, broccoli and beans, green peppers and ginger should also be used since they have a favorable *kapha* balancing effect. They are even better when consumed with *kapha* pacifying spices.

5. To aid in digestion buttermilk can be consumed along with meals and plenty of warm water should be consumed, this aids in flushing out toxins from the body.

6. Spices should have a warming effect. These can include turmeric, coriander, cumin, fenugreek and cloves can be consumed in small quantities.

The following list includes tips on lifestyle that help in balancing *kapha:*

1. To balance *kapha* one should firstly start doing something. It could mean getting physical exercise for some duration every day; it could involve mental exercising such as solving puzzles and crosswords that challenge the mind. Meeting new people and building new relationships is an inherent *kapha* characteristic

2. No meal should be skipped and there should not be any fast. This is because *kapha* digestion and metabolism both tend to be slow. Breakfast should be light; lunch should be relatively heavier in comparison to dinner which should be kept light again.

3. High intensity activities are ideal for *kapha* balancing. This could include sports that have a high intensity interval kind of workout pattern such as squash and tennis. Endurance activities such as running can also be performed.

4. Oily skin should be cleaned daily and if possible even twice a day. This will eliminate the impurities and that get accumulated in skin pores due to oily nature of skin. Shampoo should be used for hair on alternate days for the same reason. An *ayurvedic* oil massage every day in the morning can help in removing toxins that are embedded in the pores and also help increase energy level

5. Protection from damp environment should be given importance. Warm spices can be used in water that should again be heated. Steam can be taken to open up blocked pores

6. At least 30 minutes should be devoted to practice of meditation on a daily basis. It helps to balance the emotions and helps to create harmony between mind, body and soul.

7. Due to imbalance, even after long sleep of more than 10 hours one may feel tired and exhausted, as if one has not slept at all. To improve the rest quality gradually, cut out sleep during the day and at night sleep early and get up before sunrise.

Although there is no direct relation between the energy and glandular systems, yet some equivalence may be established. *Vata dosha* corresponds to the thyroid type, *pitta dosha* corresponds to adrenal type and *kapha dosha* roughly correspond to gonad type. The energy type also corresponds to the response that is shown to sensory stimulation. By understanding the energy type it becomes possible to apply the holistic practice to achieve a state of harmonious balance between mind, body and soul.

Constitutional Psychology & Somatotype

In the 1940s, William Herbert Sheldon, an American psychologist developed the theory of constitutional psychology. The aim of this system was to identify the association between different body types with temperament and psychological behavior patterns of individuals. Within the context of this theory it was hypothesized that the physique or body structure of an individual has a direct correlation with the temperament or natural behavior pattern as exhibited. The body structure is genetically pre-determined and that causes people to exhibit typical personality traits coherent with those exhibited by people with similar body structures.

This theory is based on 3 basic elements also called Somatotypes. These have been named after groups of cells also called *germinal epithelium* which are formed during the process of growth of embryo into fetus. Also referred to as germ layers these are a pronounced presence in the vertebrates. These germ layers came to be known as *mesoderm, endoderm* and *ectoderm.*

Endoderm

Endoderm is a germ layer which is made up of flattened cells initially which then become columnar in nature. It forms a predominant portion of the epithelial lining of the lungs, trachea, pharynx and the digestive tube. Mainly it forms certain parts of the colon, pancreas, stomach, liver and the intestines – predominant portion of the digestive tract.

Ectoderm

Ectoderm is the beginning of the tissues that cover the surfaces of the body. It comes out first and is responsible for the formation of nerves, pigments, connective tissue heads, mammary glands, hair and most importantly the epidermis and the central nervous system.

Mesoderm

Mesoderm is the layer that is formed between the endoderm and ectoderm. It is responsible for the skeletal structure, urinary bladder, urethra, kidney and importantly the heart, skeletal muscles and blood vessels.

On the basis of the germ layers Sheldon laid down the framework for Somatotypes. Along with a team of associates numerous college students were photographed in the nude, from the front, rear and the side. The aim was to identify regularities in the different body types. After extensive observation and subsequent analysis, the three Somatotypes or extreme body structures were defined – endomorph, mesomorph and ectomorph.

Endomorphic structure was characterized by a predominant softness and roundness throughout different parts of the body. Mesomorphic structure was a predominance of bone, lean muscle and connective tissues. Ectomorphic structure was a symbolized by fragility and linearity. However, any body type was a combination of the three Somatotypes. The representation was done on a 7 point scale from 1 to 7 where 1 is the minimum and 7 is the maximum. Therefore, a person characterized by a pure endomorphic body type was represented as 7-1-1; a pure mesomorphic body type as 1-7-1 and a pure ectomorphic body type as 1-1-7. For example, 263 means 2 (low Endomorph), 6 (high Mesomorph) and 3 (low Ectomorph). In this way one body type can be compared with another body type. A basketball player will be around 147 while a good body builder will be a 173. It does not necessarily mean that all the traits are mixed together in the particular ratio. For example, 475 may mean a heavy build of Endomorph along with musculature of Mesomorph and height of the Ectomorph which may be above average. Once this had been done, on the basis of this number representation, individual characteristics and behavioral traits were predicted.

Within the structure of the research it was believed that a person with an endomorphic body will typically be contented, affable and would be able to share feelings easily. Mesomorphs would be aggressive, bold and adventurous while ectomorphs would typically be shy, introverted, inhibited and sensitive to pain. During this empirical study observers rated individuals on these characteristics and it was found that the correlation between the body type and the characteristic behavior did exist. There were quite a few questions that were raised on the method that was followed for the study. However, subsequent studies that eliminated the issues that were raised also came out with similar results. Despite the results shown by these studies, over the years, social learning researchers have refuted the results with counter arguments. According to them, learning plays an extremely important role in this link that is observed between body types and temperament and that there is no concrete direct correlation between the two. Each particular type of body is generally associated with particular characteristic traits, which have been stereotyped. This stereotype is further reinforced through different media such as marketing & advertising campaigns, movies, theatre etc. These stereotypes are then transmitted to children from adults who are exposed to these media. The children then learn and begin to incorporate these specific traits or characteristic behavior patterns as part of their natural demeanor. It is because of this reason that typical temperaments may be observed with a specific body type that an individual has.

Typical characteristics of Somatotypes

The three main body types are – Endomorph, Mesomorph and Ectomorph. Each of these body types has specific characteristics some of them are alterable while some are not. The three body types can be modulated by body composition, which itself can be altered by specific weight management techniques. A person who is currently considered an endomorph may sometime in future begin to resemble an Ectomorph; while as age progresses a Mesomorph might begin to lose lean muscle tissue and begin to resemble an Endomorph.

Endomorph

Endomorphs are characterized by a large bone or skeletal structure and a wide waist and are usually referred to as being fat. They are predisposed to storing as well as retaining body fat. The following traits generally define an Endomorph:

- ✓ Pear shaped or round body
- ✓ Short and stocky with round head
- ✓ Wide shoulders and hips
- ✓ Wider front to back in comparison to measurements from side to side
- ✓ Lot of fat specially in the upper arms, core and thighs

Endomorphs have a tendency to gain weight very easily; however, a large portion is undesirable fat and not lean muscle. Their ability to compete in sporting activities that require an individual to be agile as well as weight bearing activities that are aerobic in nature such as running is severely restricted. Sporting activities that require pure muscular strength such as power lifting are perfect for an individual who has an endomorphic structure. Muscles especially of the upper legs – quadriceps and hamstrings are extremely strong. Along with this advantageous trait, their size is well suited, in fact ideal for sports such as rugby where bulk is crucial, provided it can be supplemented with enough power. Endomorphs also generally possess good lung capacity, making activities such as rowing suitable for them.

An endomorph should try and get rid of the excess body fat. Since their bodies are predisposed to gaining & storing a lot of fat, maintaining a healthy lifestyle is crucial. They should engage themselves in long duration, moderate intensity aerobic activity like biking and brisk walking. This will result in burning a number of calories on a daily basis, predominantly through oxidation of fat. Strength training should nevertheless be done to get a better muscle to fat ratio and thereby improving metabolism. Moderate weights at a fast training pace (extremely small rest periods between sets and exercises) should be employed while doing resistance training. Weight management system should primarily ensure a reduction in the intake of calories. It should contain frequent but small meals. By restricting the intake of simple carbohydrates and fats, a good weight management meal plan for an endomorph ensures that minimal amount of the intake is stored as body fat.

Mesomorph

Mesomorphs are characterized by wide shoulders, solid torso but narrow waist and are usually referred to as being muscular. They are invariably predisposed to increase in lean muscle tissue but not storing body fat. The following traits generally define an Mesomorph:

✓ Body is wedge shaped with a narrow waist
✓ Broad shoulders and cubical head

✓ Lean muscle tissue in arms and legs

✓ Narrow from front to back in comparison to measurement from side to side

✓ Low amount of stored body fat

A Mesomorph has a large and sturdy bone structure as well as higher mass of lean muscle, thereby providing a naturally athletic physique. Coupled with the tendency to gain lean muscle they excel in most sports because of physical characteristics such as muscular strength, speed and agility. These traits along with a good response to strength as well as cardiovascular training lay down a sound platform for body building as well. They are generally good at explosive kind of sports activities such as boxing and football.

Mesomorphs have a naturally fit body but proper exercise and diet as part of a weight management plan are essential towards maintaining this physique. Strength training should be done with moderate to heavy weights and for longer duration but with moderate rest periods between sets and exercises. Aerobic activities should be included in moderate amounts as a part of the exercise program. The metabolic rates of Mesomorphs are much faster than that of Endomorphs but slower than that of Ectomorphs. Since, Mesomorphs can gain some amount of fat slightly easily as compared to pure Ectomorphs, a good healthy weight management program is essential to maintain lean and muscular physique.

Ectomorph

Ectomorphs are characterized by long and thin limbs and are usually referred to as being slim. They are not predisposed to store fat or build muscle. The following traits generally define an Ectomorph:

✓ Thin arms & legs

✓ Hip and shoulders are narrow

✓ Chest & abdomen are narrow

✓ High forehead and a receding chin

✓ Little muscle or fat

An Ectomorph is generally slender and thin, and therefore strength and power activities & sports are not suitable for them. Lack of lean muscle tissue and consequently muscular strength puts them at a big disadvantage in sports activities that require mass. Their light frame makes them suited for long duration aerobic activities such as cycling & running as well as other activities such as gymnastics. Characteristic traits such as better thermo regulation provide them with an added advantage in endurance based sports.

It is possible that body fat in Ectomorphs drops to extremely low levels which can be dangerous to health and in case of females who participate in long duration endurance activities it can result in severe iron deficiency. Ectomorphs should concentrate on gaining weight in the form of good lean muscle tissue (some women who are too thin may also want to put on a little fat to look more feminine). Weight training should be done but not too often or for too long in each session. Workouts should be short and intense focusing on big muscle groups. Weights lifted should be moderately heavy and rest periods between sets should be longer for better recovery. Long duration aerobic activities should be kept to a minimum, to prevent undue loss of lean muscle tissue. They have an extremely fast metabolism which burns up calories very quickly. Therefore they need a huge amount of calories in order to gain weight. A high calorie diet is therefore required at the same time ensuring that low quality junk food is avoided.

Types of Body Shapes

Once we have a basic understanding of Somatotypes, we can move ahead and understand their practical application which essentially helps in defining body shape. The following is a list of different body shapes:

Male Ectomorphs

Male Ectomorphs are individuals with long and thin limbs – both arms and legs. Circumference of waist, ankle and wrist is very small. They do not gain weight and are called 'hard gainers' in common parlance. Even when they manage to gain some weight it is generally fat which is put in the abdominal region alone. They find it close to impossible to put on or gain any sort of lean muscle tissue. A big reason behind this is their extremely high metabolic rate. Despite these shortcomings, male ectomorphs are pretty good at long duration endurance activities such as biking and running.

Male Mesomorphs

Male Mesomorphs are muscular and are extremely athletic in nature. They generally have a large lean muscle mass base and this is clearly visible in their thick arms, wide chest, broad shoulders and strong legs & calves. They respond extremely well to exercise programs but in case of inactivity they tend to gain some weight also fast. It is therefore imperative the male Mesomorphs participate in regular physical activities to maintain their near perfect physiques.

Male Ecto–Mesomorphs

As the name of this body shape suggests, male ecto–mesomorphs are a combination of ectomorph and mesomorph somatotypes. Individuals in this category have a tendency to move between being extremely muscular to being extremely thin. They may have the characteristic physical traits of mesomorphs such as explained above, but they have an inclination to gain fat typically in the abdominal region of the body. Ecto-mesomorphs can increase the lean muscle tissue in their body through regular resistance training, but unlike mesomorphs they are not generally as strong and explosive in their movements.

Male Endomorphs

Male endomorphs are generally short and stocky and have a lot of fat all over the body. They are typically apple shaped with short necks and with large circumference of waist, ankles and calves. Even if they have good cardiovascular endurance capabilities, male endomorphs find it almost impossible to lose weight. As a result of which they are prone to cardiovascular as well as coronary diseases and even lifestyle diseases such as diabetes.

Female Ectomorph

Female ectomorphs are extremely slim and the measurement is extremely low for hips, shoulders, neck, ankles and calves. Like male-ectomorphs, females have an uncanny tendency to put on whatever little fat they can, in the abdominal region and hips, while the limbs still remain long and slender. Taller women within this category are slightly more athletic in nature but fail to develop any feminine characteristics without the help of intervention through a weight management program. Typically women who fall in this category have high cardiovascular endurance and are good at long duration endurance activities. Among all the categories of women their life span is invariably the longest.

Female Mesomorph

Female mesomorphs are known for their hour-glass shaped physical structure, with wide hips and shoulders but a distinctively narrow waistline. Any weight gain or loss happens proportionally in the upper body – back, shoulders and chest and the lower body – hips and thighs. Women in this category are generally good at certain athletic sports and activities.

Female Meso-endomorph

Females generally have body fat percentages in the range of 30% which is much higher than that of men. These female meso-endomorphs are much more common than their male counterparts. Females who fall in this category generally have a pear shaped body with wide hips, medium size waist and small shoulders. Such women have a tendency to look unbalances when they go even slightly out of shape. This can easily be corrected through a proper workout program.

Female Endomorphs

Women in this category have larger upper bodies in comparison to the lower half. They have an apple shaped body with large chest and abdomen but narrower hips. These women are prone to putting on weight very easily and that too visceral fat around the organs. This makes the susceptible to cardiovascular diseases and other coronary diseases. It is therefore very important for women who are female endomorphs to ensure that through a weight management system they follow a proper lifestyle which includes exercise, proper nutrition as well as enough rest.

Changes during puberty

There is a considerable change that the body undergoes during puberty. The difference between the male and the female body starts getting accentuated at this stage. These changes happen for the reproductive reasons. Inherited genetic code plays a big factor in the body shape that starts developing at this stage. The amount of lean muscle mass and the fat distribution pattern along with the skeletal structure all are influenced by the genetic make-up of the individual.

Skeletal structure

Males on an average are taller and broader in comparison to females. Analysis of body shape though, should be done after taking into consideration the difference in height. Males generally have broad shoulders coupled with wide chest. This happens as a result of testosterone influencing the widening of the rib cage. The reason behind this is that males require more oxygen for fueling the larger muscle mass that is distributed over the body. To facilitate this increased oxygen requirement there needs to be more space for the lungs to pull in more air during respiration, as a result of which expansion of the rib cage happens.

In females at this stage of puberty, widening of hips starts occurring. Estrogen which is the female sex hormone causes the widening of the pelvic girdle specifically for the purposes of childbirth. The larger and rounded pelvic structure allows the fetus head to pass through during child birth. As a result of this widening of the pelvis, the carrying angle of the elbows also increases in comparison to that of men. The sacrum is also wider and shorter and this results in the swaying of hips distinctly visible in the walking style of females. However, these characteristics cannot be stereotyped; both male and female sex hormones are present in each and every individual and the presence of the other se hormone has some effect in determining the body shape and characteristics to a certain extent.

Fat Distribution

Fat distribution plays a significant role in defining the body shape. There is a direct correlation between current fat distribution and sex hormones levels in the body. As can be expected, the skeletal structure does not change after adulthood, but the fat distribution is can be altered by modifying dietary habits and through exercise. As fat distribution changes the shape of the body itself changes visibly.

Contrary to general belief, the right amount of fat in the body is not only acceptable but in fact is necessary for optimal health. In women estrogen causes fat to be deposited in the hips, thighs and buttocks areas. Thus women generally have smaller waists but larger hips, and thus have a lower waist hip ratio in comparison to men. Women also have a much higher body fat percentage as compared to men, this is because the body is prepared for the extra energy requirements that may needed to be met during pregnancy. Post menopause though, the fat distribution in women changes and the fat starts accumulating in the abdominal region itself, as is the case with men. While estrogen promotes storage of fat in the body, testosterone reduces the fat percentage in the body by increasing the metabolic rate.

Females have mammary glands and consequently breasts which start developing after puberty; again due to the effects of estrogen in the body. Testosterone on the contrary helps men build lean muscle tissue in the body which can be enlarged through a proper exercise routine and healthy diet as part of a weight management plan.

Posture & Gait

Body shape also has a defining say in the body posture as well as gait. These play a major role in creating physical attraction. The body shape to a certain extent is representative of the sexual hormones present at that particular point in time as well as that during puberty which points towards fertility. A good body shape apart from being pleasing also implies good health.

Body Types – Effect of Exercise & Diet

As is expected, not each and every one of us is born with the dream physique of a pure mesomorph. Like in sports some people are way more talented than others and find it much easier to excel, in physical exercise too, some people are naturally gifted and find it easier to achieve and maintain a perfectly chiseled body. This is something that is build into the genetic code over which we have no control. An ectomorph might try and eat and workout really very hard but still find it difficult to add lean muscle to the body, whereas endomorphs don't seem to lose any fat which they generally have an excess of, despite following the strictest of weight management plans and the most strenuous of exercise programs.

However, this in no way means that an ectomorph will not gain weight, nor does it mean that an endomorph will not lose fat. It is just that things will be harder than what a pure mesomorph experiences. Further, generally a person is a combination of somatotypes and it is important to first understand the body type before designing a weight management plan which aims for a particular goal or outcome. Once this has been done, adherence to the program is of utmost importance; by following the guidelines over a period of time, one is bound to overcome the genetic disadvantages and achieve the fitness targets that have been set.

Ectomorph

As discussed earlier, these are people who have very little muscle and very little fat in their body. They are also referred to as 'hard gainers' because of their tendency to gain no weight at all despite consuming a heavy diet and exercising. The reason behind this is their extremely high metabolic rate, as a result of which very little storage takes place in the body. The aim is to increase weight by an increase in lean muscle, but even if the ectomorphs eat a heavy diet they put on a little fat around the abdominal region which is most undesirable. By nature too, they do not have the physical endurance and strength that may help them in achieving these goals albeit with extra effort. However, through a proper exercise program this can be altered.

Training for an ectomorph should predominantly be a heavy strength or resistance training program but the macro cycles in the program should be planned in a controlled way since they initially possess very little muscle to perform these workouts and overtraining at this initial stage may lead to injuries jeopardizing the entire program. The focus should be in learning the techniques first and then building up a little endurance and strength both muscular and cardiovascular, before ramping up the intensity. In case this is not done chances of fast burnout may occur and the person leaves the program. A gradual increase in intensity and weight needs to be incorporated as part of the program. This is important from the perspective of program efficiency as well as from the point of view of increased chances of adherence. The following points should be taken into consideration while designing the weight management program for an ectomorph:

1. Exercise duration – The duration of the workout session should not be more than an hour in any case, since the risks of overtraining ectomorphs specially is pretty high. Considering their limited endurance level, fatigue and exhaustion starts setting in earlier than usual during the session and unnecessarily pushing harder will in no way yield results. Contrarily, it only increases the chances of an injury. The goal should be to first increase stamina and then increase the intensity of the workout, perhaps, keeping the duration of workout similar.

2. Exercises – The kind of exercises that are suited for ectomorphs are multi-joint and compound exercises. The aim is to provide an extra stimulus that is responsible for pushing the body to grow further by adding lean muscle tissue. Exercises such as squats, push–ups, pull–ups etc. are extremely useful in creating this stimulus. Not only are these exercises multi-joint but are also compound in nature, involving more than one muscle group. The issue with these exercises is that a person new to strength training will find it difficult initially and may take significant time in learning these exercises. Secondly, a variety of exercises should be used to train each and every muscle group. Since, ectomorphs have very little muscle mass, they will have certain weak areas. For example, it is important to train the entire triceps group through a variety of exercises so that the person may also be able to perform push–ups efficiently. If the triceps are left untrained, then the major muscle group while doing push–ups, chest muscles in this case do not fatigue, but the smaller

supporting muscle, in this case triceps reaches exhaustion. Hence, the exercise no longer remains efficient to train the pectorals. It is therefore crucial to train all muscle groups of the body.

3. Sets – Due to limited lean muscle tissue in the body, the number of sets per exercise should be limited. Rather a variety of exercises should be chosen for the workout session. For each muscle group and at each stage of development of the group, a certain number of sets per exercise is ideal. Once the number of sets crosses this benefits from these sets starts diminishing as well. Generally at the initial stage of the program, not more than 2 to 3 sets per exercise should be performed for each exercise.

4. Repetitions – This refers to the number of times a movement is performed in each set. The goal of any strength training program for an ectomorph is to increase lean muscle mass, this can happen through a process called hypertrophy. For hypertrophy to occur, the number of repetitions per set should be limited between 9 to 12 counts. The number of repetitions has a direct relationship with the resistance or load that is lifted for the exercise. Greater number of repetitions means lower resistance and lesser number of repetitions means that a higher resistance can be chosen. For example, an individual who is performing squats and is able to lift 100 lbs. for 12 repetitions, will be able to lift 150 lbs. in case he or she needs to perform only 6 repetitions whereas the load will go down to 75 lbs. in case the number of repetitions increases to 18. By increasing the repetitions and consequently reducing load, an endurance workout is performed. By decreasing the repetitions and consequently increasing the load a strength workout is performed. The goal for an ectomorph is gain in size or hypertrophy; this can be achieved with around 9 to 12 repetitions per set.

5. Rest between sets – Whenever an exercise is performed energy utilized is in the form of a molecule called ATP or Adenosine Tri Phosphate. This is the only energy molecule in

the body that the muscles can utilize to perform work. Metabolism of energy molecules such as carbohydrates, fats and proteins yields ATP which is then utilized. Limited amount of ATP can be stored in the working muscles therefore as we perform more and more work, ATP needs to be generated. For hypertrophy to take place, rest period between sets should be limited to 45 seconds.

6. Resistance training techniques – Simple linear general training should be performed at the initial stage. This means that in a sequential manner, 2 to 3 sets of each exercise should be performed taking into account the right number of repetitions and the appropriate rest period between the sets. Once a couple of months have passed and the person has learnt the correct techniques, new training protocols such as eccentric training, compound training, tri–sets, rest & pause and super sets can be incorporated as part of the workout. Initially however, things should be kept simple and manageable.

7. Calorie count – An ideal target is a gain of around 1 to 2 lbs. of lean mass per week. To do this, an energy excess of around 750 calories per day needs to be achieved. This energy excess shall be utilized in repair and growth of the muscle tissue that has been utilized during workout. In the absence of any workout, it starts getting stored as fat. Therefore, workout and diet go together in helping an individual achieve his or her fitness goals.

8. Frequency of meals – Ectomorphs have a very high metabolic rate, therefore it is important that the body is fuelled on a regular basis. By performing high intensity exercise, the requirement of the body goes up. In case adequate energy is not provided at the correct time, the body starts utilizing resources from within. This is not desirable since the goal is weight gain and we do not want any loss of weight happening due to inadequate energy being provided to the body. It is therefore important to consume meals every two to three hours so that the body is fuelled at the correct rate to enhance growth.

9. Meal Content – The dietary breakup should be such that all macro nutrients as well as micro nutrients are made available in sufficient quantities. A diet in which the amount of calories derived from carbohydrates is 45%, from proteins is 35% and that from fats is 20% is ideal. A few alterations can be made within this structure to suit individual needs.

10. Pre & Post workout meals – These are extremely important meals of the day and the efficiency of a workout session can double if the right kind of nutrition is made available to the body prior to, during and after the workout. In an ectomorph, the goal is to increase weight by utilizing resources from outside to fuel the requirements of the body. Lesser the dependence on internal sources better it is. Prior to the workout, a combination of complex carbohydrates with some protein source is ideal. This will ensure that the body is gradually provided energy over the duration of the workout. In case an energy deficit is experienced during the workout then during the next workout, pre-workout meal content could be ramped up with an increased amount of carbohydrates. Post workout meal is important since this is when the muscle tissues open up a kind of anabolic or growth window. A combination of simple sugars such as glucose & fructose along with fast acting proteins such as whey seems ideal for the purpose. The insulin spike experienced as a result of glucose entering the blood stream will help in the pushing glycogen into the muscles. Eating at regular intervals after this will provide the right kind of environment for the muscles to grow.

11. Types of food – Apart from the anabolic phase, it is important to consume slow metabolizing foods such as complex carbohydrates and slow acting proteins. This will ensure that storage by conversion into fat is avoided when the body does not require energy at that fast rate. At the same time the energy as well as growth requirements of the body are met.

Along with the right kind of diet and exercise as part of a weight management plan ectomorphs should rest appropriately, since the muscles need time to recover from the strain they have been put under. A combination of these three components of fitness will lead to healthy weight gain in the long duration.

Mesomorphs

Mesomorphs possess the ideal body type. They are generally muscular and athletic with little amount of fat in the body. In case this is not the case, and dude to some reason they have put on fat, still, their natural predisposition is towards losing fat and increasing lean muscle tissue in the body. The genetic build up is such that it is inclined towards a muscular physique with broad shoulders and wider side to side measurement in comparison to front to back measurements. The following points should be taken into consideration while designing a weight management program for a mesomorph:

1. Duration of exercise – Since they possess a physical structure that can endure higher intensities, duration of exercise should generally be an hour but it can go up on certain days which may be kept for heavy endurance training. Even Mesomorphs though can be new to exercise and strength training in particular. It is important to appreciate this fact and go slow in the initial stages of the program. Gradually, the intensity can be increased to higher levels since the body is suited to perform under these circumstances. Understanding the techniques first should be given priority before ramping up the volume & load. It is also important to understand the limits of the body and a number of Mesomorphs commit the mistake of overtraining and putting the body under undue stress.

2. Exercises – Mesomorphs should perform a combination of all exercises. Their workouts in general should cover all aspects of fitness – muscular strength, muscular endurance, cardiovascular endurance and flexibility. There can be specific training goals such as increasing lean mass for bigger physique or improving cardiovascular endurance for long distance running. In these situations workout should be goal specific and should predominantly work towards better performance in that respect, however, other aspect of fitness

should also be given due importance for optimal health. A combination of different strength training exercises should be chose. These should include single as well as multi-joint exercises, compound as well as isolated movements. Even for improving cardiovascular endurance a combination of workouts should be chosen such as running, swimming, biking etc. These different exercises though working on cardiovascular endurance utilize different muscle groups and add variety in a manner such that overall fitness of the individual improves.

3. Sets – General training programs should include workout days which concentrate on building up of muscular strength, increasing muscular endurance as well as sessions for hypertrophy. Such a well rounded macro plan will ensure a good balance. When the goal is hypertrophy the number of sets should increase as increased volume of workout is the requirement. When gaining strength is the goal, number of sets can be moderate to high, while when endurance is the goal, the number of sets per exercise should be moderate.

4. Repetitions – The number of repetitions per set and consequently the resistance or load should also vary depending on the purpose of the workout session. For strength gains the number of repetitions per set is small, in the range of 4 to 6 and load is higher, for hypertrophy number of repetitions is moderate – 9 to 12, and so is the load, and for muscular endurance the number of repetitions is high – 16 to 18 and even more, and load or resistance comes down considerably.

5. Rest between sets – The rest between sets should be kept at around 45 seconds to 1 minute, unless workout is being performed for strength gains. In this case, the rest period can go up to 3 minutes. The reason behind this is that the exercising muscle needs to recover and enough ATP needs to be present in the muscle to perform the exercise for the next set.

6. Training techniques – Unlike ectomorphs and endomorphs, mesomorphs should incorporate a lot of variety in their workouts. Once the technique of training and method or pos-

ture for each exercise being performed has been learnt, Mesomorphs should incorporate not only different exercises but also different routines and workout patterns. This ensures that a different stimulus is being provided to the body in each workout and therefore the body improves further over a period of time.

7. Calorie count – Depending on the goal of the individual mesomorph, calorie count can vary. In case a weight gain is desired then energy excess needs to be achieved while if weight loss is desired then energy deficit needs to be created. In general, an excess or a deficit of around 500 calories per day is ideal depending on the goal. This will lead to a weight difference of around 1 to 2 lbs. per week which is a healthy target.

8. Meal frequency – A 6 meal program including pre & post workout meals ensures that the body is provided energy and nutrition when it requires it. It then has no need to store any of this extra energy in the body.

9. Meal content – A balanced nutrition program with the right macro nutrient as well as micro nutrients and anti-oxidants is desired. The percentage of calories from can be in the following ratio: 55–60% from carbohydrates, 15–20% from proteins and 20–25% from fats. A variety of foods should be consumed so that all the necessary vitamins & proteins are made available to the body in the right quantities.

10. Pre & Post workout meals – Pre-workout meal should be such that there is sufficient energy in the body to perform exercises at the intensity that is desired. Post workout meal should be such that it provides ample fuel immediately for growth. As in other cases, the meal content and quantity depends on the goal of the program. Weight loss goals will entail meal patterns such that resources such as stored glycogen and fat are utilized from within the body, while weight gain goals will need meals such that enough energy as well as amino acids from protein break down is made available through a proper diet all throughout the day and specifically immediately after exercise session.

The workout and diet pattern for Mesomorphs is completely dependent on the goal. Since, Mesomorphs in general can have variety of workout objectives, therefore it is important to first understand those goals and then design an appropriate program. Once those goals are achieved Mesomorphs enter maintenance phase which requires a well rounded and balanced workout routine as well as diet program.

Endomorphs

Endomorphs have a large skeletal structure and are predisposed to storing a lot of fat all over the body. They have wide shoulders as well as hips and accumulate lot of fat in the upper arms, thighs as well as abdominal region. Endomorphs have a tendency to gain weight very easily; however, a large portion is undesirable fat and not lean muscle. The program goal for endomorphs is to reduce the body fat percentage drastically. In case of endomorphs who have lost this fat, the aim is them to maintain this at the same time to try and increase lean muscle mass. The following points should be taken into consideration while designing a weight management program for a mesomorph:

1. Duration of exercise – The maximum duration of exercise for endomorphs should be around an hour. There is a tendency to overdo cardiovascular workouts for long durations above the one hour mark. However, this leads to unnecessary loss of lean muscle tissue. There are ways and methods which when applied properly can help in lose fat at the same time prevent the loss of lean muscle tissue to a certain extent. As is the case with other body types the intensity of workouts should increase only gradually once techniques and correct methods to perform exercises have been learnt.

2. Exercises – Endomorphs should perform exercises covering all aspects of fitness but the main attention is towards burning calories through cardiovascular endurance as well as strength training workouts. Aerobic activities such as jogging, swimming, cycling are appropriate cardiovascular workouts. In case the individual is extremely obese, then non–impact activities such as cycling on a recumbent bike

are more suitable since the load on the knees is limited.

It is also important to understand the concept of heart rate in this regard. Whenever a person exercises the heart rate increases from that at rest. The maximum heart rate of a person is age dependent. Thus, the heart rate can vary between these two levels – resting heart rate and maximum heart rate. The difference between the two is called the heart rate reserve. When a person works out at an intensity corresponding to 40 to 50% of the heart rate reserve then the activity is aerobic in nature. This means that the production of energy happens by metabolism in the presence of oxygen. This is important since fat can be burned only through aerobic methods. As the intensity increases the process becomes anaerobic and fat will no longer be used as the primary source of energy. Thus, exercises should be performed at a moderate intensity to burn fat. This is extremely important to build into the exercise program.

Further, endomorphs should try and burn calories through resistance training workouts as well. Multi-joint compound movements are preferred since they burn more number of calories in comparison to isolated exercises. Also, free weight exercises are preferred in comparison to working out on machines. The reason behind this is that the balance and coordination that is required for free weight exercises require significantly higher neuro-muscular coordination. This means a greater effort and higher number of calories being burnt in the process as well.

3. Sets – The primary training goal of endomorphs is to burn calories and to utilize the stored fat in the body for the purpose. Cardiovascular workouts should be performed for at least 20 to 30 minutes and this can go up as endurance increases and the heart rate continues to remain at a moderate level even at higher intensities and after long durations. For resistance training, the number of sets can be 3 per exercise in such a way that all body parts are worked out over the course of the week. Since the choice of exercises are generally compound in nature that utilize many muscle groups,

the chance of leaving out a particular muscle is generally low, but still care should be taken to avoid this.

4. Repetitions – The number of repetitions per set should be kept high since the effort is to burn more calories. This can be from 12 – 15 repetitions per set.

5. Rest between sets – The rest between sets should be kept at around 30 – 45 seconds. In such a situation the heart rate remains elevated even during resistance training workouts and mimics a cardiovascular workout. When the heart rate remains elevated it leads to burning more number of calories throughout the exercise session.

6. Training techniques – Endomorphs can incorporate numerous techniques and workout principles. Ideal ones are those in which exercises are performed back to back with minimal rest between sets. For example, circuit training is a workout principle in which a set of around 10 – 12 exercises of various muscle groups are performed for a specific number of repetitions without rest between exercises. A person moves from one station to another immediately and does not rest until the entire circuit is completed. Such workouts keep the heart rate at an elevated level, helping the body to burn fat consistently.

7. Calorie count – This particular parameter is most important for endomorphs. The goal is to lose approximately 2 lbs. of fat every week on a continuous basis. This means an energy deficit of around 1,000 calories needs to be created on a daily basis. Thus the intake needs to be carefully measured and monitored.

8. Meal frequency – A high frequency low calorie meal plan is ideal for endomorphs. The body does not require huge amounts of energy at any time during the day. Heavy meals will lead to utilization of a part of the calories ingested and storage as fat of the remaining amount. A weight management diet plan such as 6 meal plan ensures that the body gets only what it requires and when it requires it. There is no storage since there is no excess left after the calories from that meal have been utilized.

9. Meal content – Contrary to numerous myths and popular weight loss diet plans, a balanced nutritious diet is correct for even endomorphs trying to lose weight. The percentage of calories can be in the following ratio – 50–55% from carbohydrates, 20–25% from proteins and 20–25% from fats. A variety of foods should be included in the diet plan so that all the essential micro-nutrients are available for the smooth functioning of the body.

10. Pre & Post workout meals – Pre-workout meal can include a small complex carbohydrate snack that ensures that there is energy in the body to perform the workout. Working out on an empty stomach has numerous issues associated with it and therefore should be avoided. Post workout meal should also consist of complex carbohydrates along with fast acting protein. This means that even after workout when the heart rate remains elevated due to principles like EPOC (excess post-exercise oxygen consumption) the body uses the stored reserves such as body fat for fulfilling this energy requirement.

Endomorphs should be mindful that too much of a cardiovascular workout is not performed and that too at high intensities. The reason for this is that although there will be considerable loss of weight, it will involve loss of lean muscle tissue as well. This situation is not desirable and should be avoided. In most cases, however, there is some amount of muscle loss that happens and once endomorphs have lost the excess fat in the body, the weight management plan should focus on recovering the lost lean muscle tissue in the process.

Irrespective of the type of body that an individual possesses it is possible through a combination of proper diet, exercise and rest to alter the characteristics inherent with the body type. The body type is built into our genetic structure, but that does not mean that the traits associated with the body type are beyond our control. It may require significant amount of effort but it is possible for an endomorph to lose excess fat, and it is possible for an ectomorph to gain lean muscle tissue.

Body goals diary

_____

_____

_____

_____

_____

_____

_____

_____

_____

_____

_____

_____

_____

_____

Body goals diary

_____

_____

_____

_____

_____

_____

_____

_____

_____

_____

_____

_____

_____

Body goals diary

_____

_____

_____

_____

_____

_____

_____

_____

_____

_____

_____

_____

_____

_____

_____

Body goals diary

_____

_____

_____

_____

_____

_____

_____

_____

_____

_____

_____

_____

_____

_____

Body goals diary

_____

_____

_____

_____

_____

_____

_____

_____

_____

_____

_____

_____

_____

_____

Body goals diary

_____

_____

_____

_____

_____

_____

_____

_____

_____

_____

_____

_____

_____

Body goals diary

_____

_____

_____

_____

_____

_____

_____

_____

_____

_____

_____

_____

_____

_____

_____

Body goals diary

_____

_____

_____

_____

_____

_____

_____

_____

_____

_____

_____

_____

_____

Body goals diary

_____

_____

_____

_____

_____

_____

_____

_____

_____

_____

_____

_____

_____

_____

Body goals diary

_____

_____

_____

_____

_____

_____

_____

_____

_____

_____

_____

_____

_____

_____

Body goals diary

_____

_____

_____

_____

_____

_____

_____

_____

_____

_____

_____

_____

_____

Body goals diary

_____

_____

_____

_____

_____

_____

_____

_____

_____

_____

_____

_____

_____

Body goals diary

_____

_____

_____

_____

_____

_____

_____

_____

_____

_____

_____

_____

_____

_____

Body goals diary

_____

_____

_____

_____

_____

_____

_____

_____

_____

_____

_____

_____

_____

Body goals diary

_____

_____

_____

_____

_____

_____

_____

_____

_____

_____

_____

_____

_____

_____

Body goals diary

_____

_____

_____

_____

_____

_____

_____

_____

_____

_____

_____

_____

_____

Body goals diary

_____

_____

_____

_____

_____

_____

_____

_____

_____

_____

_____

_____

_____

_____

Body goals diary

_____

_____

_____

_____

_____

_____

_____

_____

_____

_____

_____

_____

_____

_____

Body goals diary

_____

_____

_____

_____

_____

_____

_____

_____

_____

_____

_____

_____

_____

_____

Body goals diary

_____

_____

_____

_____

_____

_____

_____

_____

_____

_____

_____

_____

About the author

C. T. Pam is not a physician, rather she is a regular person who has explored many avenues of eating healthy and finding a healthy lifestyle balance. After a car accident in 2010 left her unable to continue running, she found a work-life balance that has helped her maintain a healthy lifestyle. C. T. Pam has a B.A. in Political Science and Studio Art, an MBA with a entrepreneurship concentration and is currently pursuing a doctoral degree with a research focus in Entrepreneurship.

Book description

This book includes sound advice and facts regarding

- Introduction to weight management
- Choosing meal portions

While this book doesn't intend to tell the reader the best way to lead a healthy lifestyle, the author advises the reader to take away items that he or she can realistically achieve. You won't lose 50 pounds overnight, and you will have an opportunity to explore options that might benefit your physical, emotional and lifestyle needs. This book includes pages for the reader to record their goals and progress.

Volume 1 is an excerpt from Adopting a healthy lifestyle (1-884711-34-0)

Also available from Innovative Publishers

Introduction to the Paleo diet. (978-1884711466)

Introduction to the Paleo diet + 200 recipes (1884711820)

Love is... (978-1884711138)

Extreme Betrayal (978-1884711084)

Beware the Bumble Bee (978-1884711091)

Doing business with the U. S. government (978-1884711107)

Visit http://innovative-publishers.com for ordering information

Find us online @

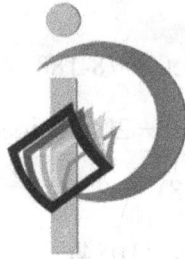

Innovative Publishers

InnovaPub

www.innovative-publishers.com

pub@innovative-publishers.com

http://innovativepublishers.blogspot.com/

http://www.facebook.com/InnovativePublishers

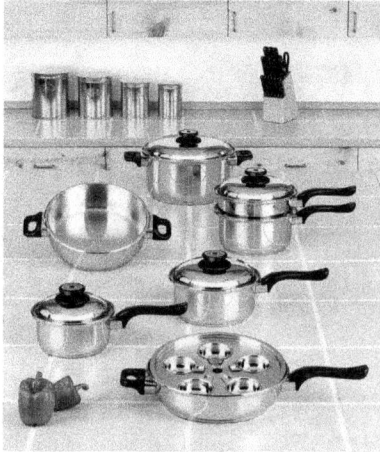

World's Finest™ 7-Ply Steam Control™ 17pc T304 Stainless Steel Cookware Set

Each piece is constructed of extra-heavy stainless steel and guaranteed to last a lifetime. Steam control valves make "waterless" cooking easy and the 7-ply construction spreads heat quickly and evenly, allowing one stack to cook. Cookware is also equipped with superbly styled phenolic handles resistant to heat, cold and detergents. Comes with a limited lifetime warranty. White box.

Suggested Retail Price : $2195.00

Item Number : GGKT17ULTRA

Set Contents

- 1.7Qt Covered Saucepan
- 2.5Qt Covered Saucepan
- 3.2Qt Covered Saucepan
- 7.5Qt Covered Roaster
- 11-3/8" Skillet, Double Boiler Unit With Capsule Bottom That You Can Also Use As An Extra 3Qt Saucepan
- 5 Egg Cups
- 5 Hole Utility Rack And High Dome Cover With Capsule Bottom So You Can Use As A Frypan
- Cover Fits Skillet Or Roaster

Features

- Extra-Heavy Stainless Steel Construction
- Heat-Resistant Phenolic Handles
- 7-Ply Construction

Limited Lifetime Warranty

» Estimated Case Weight : 36.55 Lbs.

Advertisement

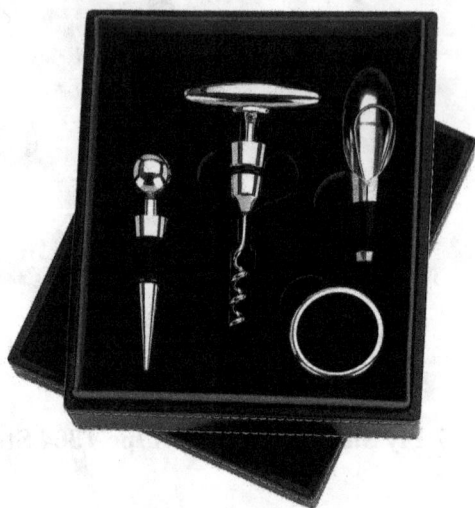

Wyndham House™ 4pc Wine Set in Storage Case

Wyndham House™ wine sets are a great compliment to any home bar, and are sure to add to the ease and elegance of wine presentations. Includes stainless steel wine spout, stainless steel wine ring, zinc alloy screw opener, and zinc alloy wine stopper. All enclosed in a 6-3/8" x 5-5/8" x 2-1/4" faux leather case.

Suggested Retail Price : $32.95

Next Ship Date : 01/05/2013

Item Number : GGKTWINE4

Features

- Stainless Steel Wine Spout
- Stainless Steel Wine Ring
- Zinc Alloy Screw Opener
- Zinc Alloy Wine Stopper
- 6-3/8" X 5-5/8" X 2-1/4" Faux Leather Case

Shipping Details

» Estimated Piece Weight : 1.10 Lbs.

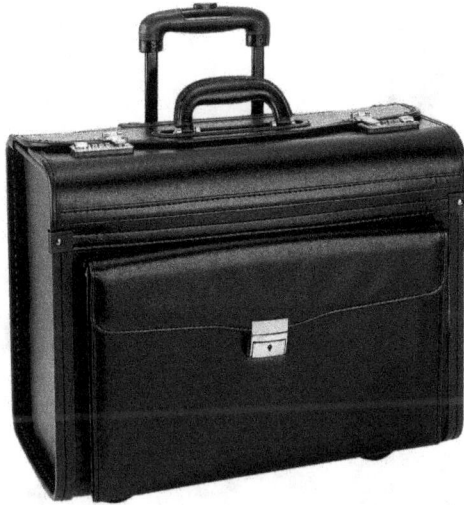

Embassy™ Sample/Pilot Case with Aluminum Trolley

Features PVC matte black exterior, rolling wheels, gunmetal combination locks, carrying handle, 2 exterior pockets, interior dividers, interior pockets, and pen holders. Measures 19" x 14" x 9".

Suggested Retail Price : $233.95

Number : BCPILOT3

Features

- Pvc Matte Black Exterior
- Rolling Wheels
- Gunmetal Combination Locks
- Carrying Handle
- 2 Exterior Side Pockets
- Interior Dividers & Pockets
- Pen Holders
- Measures 18" X 13" X 8"

Shipping Details

» Estimated Piece Weight : 8.70 Lbs.

To order products, go to the Innovative Publishers website and click Client specials. Clients receive up to 70% off the suggested retail price.

www.ingramcontent.com/pod-product-compliance
Lightning Source LLC
Chambersburg PA
CBHW050551280326
41933CB00011B/1798